The Fast Ketogenic Diet Recipe Book

Fit and Savory Recipes to Burn Fat and eating and Living Well Everyday

Michelle Lewis

Contents

Avocado chaffle

Preparation time: 5 minutes

Cooking time: 8 minutes

Servings: 1

Ingredients

Big spray of avocado oil or olive oil/coconut oil large waffle iron

2 oz thinly sliced cheese (cheddar or co lby work best)

1 large egg whisked small waffle iron (single waffle Ingredients)

1 oz thinly sliced cheese (cheddar or colby work best)

1/3 large egg whisked

Directions:

Sprinkle avocado oil first, then cover the bottom of your hot w. (i cut mine into triangles because i've got a bigger waffle iron) whisk 1 egg together (if you're using a mini waffle iron, use just 1/3 on an egg) and pour over. Place another layer of thin-sliced cheese on top to ensure that you are completely coated. Fry absolutely until the waffle iron can be lifted without the cheese sticking-depending on your waffle iron usually takes around 6-8 minutes.

Nutritional value: Calories 300

Calories from fat 221 Fat 24.5g38%

Saturated fat 12.3g77% Carbohydrates 2g1%

Protein 19g38%

Original chaffle

Preparation   time: 5   minutes

Cooking   time: 5   minutes

Servings: 1

Ingredients

2 eggs

1 cup cheddar cheese

Directions:

Heat mini waffle maker (takes 30 seconds).

Whisk 2 eggs and 1 cup cheese in a small bowl.

Add the mixture to the waffle maker and spell for 2-3 minutes.

This mixture makes two chaffles.

Nutritional value

Yield: 2 Servings, 1 serving: 1 oriental chaffle serving size: calories: 168, total carbohydrates: 1g, fiber: 0g, net carbohydrates: 1g, total fat: 13g, protein: 12g

Broccoli & cheddar

Ketogenic waffles

Preparation time: 5 minutes

Cooking time: 5 *minutes*

Servings: 1

Ingredients:

⅓ raw broccoli, finely chopped 20 g

¼ cup cheddar cheese, shredded 28g

1 egg

1/2 teaspoon garlic powder

1/2 tsp dried onion

Salt and pepper flavor

Cooking spray

Directions:

To reach the temperature, insert a waffle iron.

Beat the egg with a fork in a small bowl.

Fold in broccoli, cheese, powdered garlic, onions, salt, pepper.

Use Cooking spray as soon as the waffle iron is ready (if needed) and add the egg mixture. Cover well waffle iron and apply heat till the light indicates that one cycle is complete.

Close the lid again and cook for another period.

When finished, gently remove the waffle iron with a tongue or fork.

Enjoy! Enjoy! Servings with honey, sour cream, pasture and other sauces.

Note: this recipe makes one or two mini waffles at full size.

Sprinkle with crushed cheddar cheese before and after spreading the egg mixture.

Nutritional value

Servings: 1 serving calories: 125kcal carbohydrates: 4g protein: 7g fat: 9g fiber: 1g

Maple cream cheese icing

Preparation	time:	5	minutes
Cooking	time:	10	*minutes*

Servings: 5

Ingredients:

4 oz cream cheese

1/2 cup heavy cream

1/4 cup lacanto maple flavor syrup

1 teaspoon of vanilla essence

1/4 teaspoon of cinnamon

Directions

combine softened cream cheese and all other Ingredients in a blender start with a pulse to combine before blending until smooth nutritional value

Servings:		1	oz
calories:			70kcal
carbohydrates:			1g
protein:			1g
fat:			7g
saturated	fat:		4g
cholesterol:			24mg
sodium:			34mg

potassium:		20mg
fiber:		1g
|	calcium:	16mg
iron: 1mg		

Pumpkin pecan chaffle

Preparation time: 5 minutes

Cooking time: 10 minutes total ti me: 15 minutes

Servings: 5

Ingredients:1 egg

1/2 cup of mozzarella cheese grated

1 tablespoon pumpkin puree

1/2 teaspoon pumpkin spice

1 teaspoon erythritol low carb sweetener

2 tablespoons almond flour

2 tablespoons of minced toast

Directions

turn on the waffle maker and graze slightly (provides a light olive oil spray). Beat the eggs in the bowl. Remove mozzarella cheese, pumpkin, almond flour, pumpkin and erythritol seasonings and mix well spoon the dough evenly into the waffle maker with a spoon (repeat if you have a small waffle maker that uses half of the mixture to make the waffle) close the lid and cook for 5 minutes. Use whipped cream or low carb caramel sauce with tongs and cut fried waffles. Maybe some pecan nuts note net carbohydrates are calculated by subtracting the number of fibers from the total number of carbohydrates. Carbohydrates remove alcohol from starch.

Nutritional value: calories: 210kcal carbohydrates: 4.6g protein: 11g fat: 17g fiber: 1.7g

Pumpkin chaffle churros

Preparation time: 5 minutes

Cooking time: 20 *minutes*

Servings: 3

Ingredients: 1 cup mozzarella cheese

1 egg 1/4 cup pumpkin puree

1/4 cup coconut flour

2 tbsp lacant golden monk fruit sweetener

1 teaspoon of vanilla essence

1 tsp baking powder

1/2 tsp pumpkin spice seasoning

1/8 teaspoon of real salt

Churro cinnamon monk fruit topping

1 tbsp cinnamon ground

Lakant golden monk fruit sweetener 1 tbsp

Directions

put all Ingredients in a mixing bowl, then pour the mixture into a piping bag cut the chips from the piping bag and pipe the pumpkin chaffle mixture into each slot of the churro maker cook until brown (about 4 minutes) nutritional value

Calories: 98kcal carbohydrates: 6g protein: 6g fat: 6g saturated fat: 3g cholesterol: 42mg sodium: 188mg potassium: 130mg fiber: 3g sugar: 1g vitamin a: 1755iu vitamin c: 1mg calcium: 150mg iron: 1mg

Cinnamon roll chaffles with cream cheese frosting

Preparation time: 5 minutes

Cooking time: 5 *minutes*

Servings: 1

Ingredients:

1 tbsp cream cheese, tender (or an alternative to sour cream or ricotta cheese)

One large egg

1 teaspoon of melted butter

2 tablespoons almond flour (or 1 tablespoon coconut powder)

1/4 teaspoon baking powder

1 teaspoon ground cinnamon

1/2 teaspoon vanilla extract

1/4 teaspoon of cinnamon extract (or add 1/2 teaspoon of cinnamon)

6-8 drops of lakanto monkfruit extract to taste (or 2 teaspoons of granular erythritol)

Cream cheese frosting Ingredients:

1 oz cream cheese, softened

2 teaspoons powdered erythritol or taste

1 teaspoon of vanilla essence

1-2 tablespoons of heavy cream

Directions

 preheat a waffle maker with a mini 4. (if you use a regular size waffle maker, double or triple the recipe.) Mix all the Ingredients until a smooth batter form. (if necessary, microwave the cold cream cheese for about 5-8 seconds to soften before adding the remaining Ingredients.) Divide the batter into two and cook each cake for 4 minutes until well browned and crispy. Two mini 4 "chaffles are made from this recipe.

Whisk together the whole frosting components in a small bowl and add enough heavy cream to achieve the desired consistency of spreading. Spread the frosting on the warm chaffles and add extra cinnamon to sprinkle. Enjoy! Enjoy!

Nutritional value

408 calories, 9.3 g

Carbohydrate (2.8 g dietary fiber, 2.3 g sugars)

34.8 g total fat (16.8 g saturated fat, 0 g trans-fat)

271 mg cholesterol

352 mg sodium

202 mg calcium

192 mg potassium

932 mg vit a

2 mg iron

12.4 g protein.

Net carbs per serving: 6.5 grams

Ketogenic pumpkin
cheesecake chaffle

Preparation	time:	2	minutes
Cooking	time:	4	*minutes*

Servings: 2

Ingredients: pumpkin chaffle

1 egg

1/2 cup mozzarella cheese

1 1/2 tbsp pumpkin puree (100% pumpkin)

1 tablespoon almond flour

1 tbsp. Of la canto golden sweetener or sweetener choice

2 tsp heavy cream

1 teaspoon cream cheese

1/2 tsp pumpkin spice

1/2 teaspoon baking powder

1/2 teaspoon vanilla

1 teaspoon chocolate zero maple syrup or 1/8 teaspoon maple extract

Filling

2 tablespoons cream cheese

1 tablespoon lakant powder sweetener

1/4 teaspoon of vanilla essence

Directions

preheat mini waffle maker in a small bowl, mix all chaffle Ingredients.

Pour half of the chaffle mixture into the center of the waffle iron. Cook for 3-5 minutes.

Carefully remove and repeat the second chaffle. While making the filling, set it to the crunchy side.

With a whisk or fork, mix all the matte Ingredients together. Add a frost between the two chaffles. Pleasant!

Optional: add whipped cream top, crushed pecans, chocolate zero maple syrup and more.

Nutritional value

Calories: 204.25

Total fat: 15.25g

Carbohydrates: 3.3g

Net carbohydrates: 2.65g

Fiber: 0.65g

Protein: 12.05g

Ketogenic chaffle stuffing

Preparation time: 20 minutes

Cooking time: 40 minutes

Servings: 4

Ingredients

Basic chaffle Ingredients

1/2 cup cheese mozzarella, cheddar cheese, or a combination of both

2 eggs

1/4 teaspoon of garlic powder

1/2 teaspoon onion powder

1/2 teaspoon dried chicken seasoning

1/4 teaspoon salt

1/4 teaspoon pepper

Ingredients for filling

1 diced onion

2 celery stems

4 oz mushrooms diced

4 cups of butter for sauteing

3 eggs

Directions:

First, make a chaffle. This recipe makes four mini-chaffles.

Preheat mini waffle iron.

Preheat oven to 350f

In a medium bowl, mix the chaffle Ingredients.

Pour 1/4 of the mixture into a mini waffle maker and cook each chaffle for about 4 minutes each.

When they are all cooked, set aside.

In a small skillet, fry the onions, celery and mushrooms until soft.

In a separate bowl, split the chaffle into small pieces and add sauteed vegetables and three eggs. Mix until the Ingredients are completely bonded.

Add the mixture of fillings to a small casserole dish (about 4x4) and bake at 350 degrees for about 30-40 minutes.

Note

(make four chaffles)

Nutritional value

Calories 229

% daily value*

Total fat 17.6g 27%

Cholesterol 265.6mg 89%

Sodium 350mg 15%

Total carbohydrate 4.6g 2%

Dietary fiber 1.1g 5%

Sugars 2g

Protein 13.7g 27%

Vitamin a 217.2μg 14%

Vitamin c 2.4mg 4%

Ketogenic sausage ball chaffle

Preparation time: 5 minutes

Cooking time: 3 minutes

Servings: 2

Ingredients

1-pound bulk italian sausage

1 cup almond flour

2 teaspoons baking powder

1 cup shredded cheddar cheese

1/4 cup grated parmesan cheese

1 egg, or if you are allergic to eggs, you can use flax eggs

Directions:

Heat the maker of mini waffles to average.

Put all the Ingredients in a big bowl and combine well by hand.

Place a paper plate to trap any drops under the waffle maker.

In a hot waffle maker, spoon a 3-t blend.

Cook for a total of 3 minutes. Switch over and cook to get a crisp look for another 2 minutes.

Nutritional value

Garlic parmesan chaffle:

Preparation time: 7 minutes

Cooking time: 7 *minutes*

Servings: 2

Ingredients: 1/2 tsp italian seasoning

1/2 cup mozzarella cheese (shredded)

1/3 cup grated parmesan cheese

One large egg

1 piece of garlic (chopped or used 1/2 to reduce the flavor of garlic)

1/4 teaspoon baking powder (optional)

Directions

Preheat the waffle iron for about 5 minutes until hot. If your recipe includes cream cheese, put it in a bowl first. Gently heat in a microwave (15-30 seconds) or double boiler until soft and stir. Stir all remaining Ingredients (except toppings, if any). Pour a sufficient amount of chaffle dough into the waffle maker and cover the surface firmly. (for a normal waffle maker, about 1/2 cup, for a mini waffle maker, about 1/4 cup.) Cook for about 3-4 minutes until brown and crisp. Carefully remove the chaffle from the waffle maker and set aside for a crisp noise. (cooling is important for the texture!) If there is any dough, repeat with the remaining dough.

Nutrition: Calories 208 16g fat

11g protein 4g total carbs

2g pure carbohydrate Fiber2g Sugar 0g

Traditional Ketogenic
low carb chaffle

Preparation time: 5 minutes

Cooking time: 8 *minutes*

Servings: 1

Ingredients:

1 egg

1/2 cup shredded cheddar cheese

Directions

 turn on or plug in the waffle maker, heat and grease both sides.

After breaking the eggs in a small bowl, add 1/2 cup of cheddar cheese and mix.

Pour half of the dough into the waffle maker and close the top.

Cook for 3-4 minutes or until the desired degree of baking is achieved.

Carefully remove from the waffle maker and leave for 2-3 minutes to give time to crisp.

Follow the instructions again to make a second chaffle.

This recipe of traditional chaffle makes a great sandwich.

Nutrition: Calories: 291kcal

carbohydrates: 1g protein: 20g fat: 23g

saturated fat: 13g cholesterol: 223mg

sodium: 413mg potassium: 116mg

sugar: 1g iron: 1mg

Chicken zinger chaffle

Preparation time: 15 min

Cooking time: 15 min

Servings: 2

Ingredients

1 chicken breast, cut into 2 pieces

1/2 cup coconut flour

1/4 cup finely grated parmesan

1 tsp. Paprika

1/2 tsp. Garlic powder

1/2 tsp. Onion powder

1 tsp. Salt& pepper

1 egg beaten

Avocado oil for frying

Lettuce leaves

Bbq sauce

Chaffle Ingredients

4 oz. Cheese

2 whole eggs

2 oz. Almond flour

1/4 cup almond flour

1 tsp baking powder

Directions

Mix together chaffle Ingredients in a bowl.

Pour the chaffle batter in preheated greased square chaffle maker.

Cook chaffles for about 2-3 minutes until cooked through.

Make 4 square chaffles from this batter.

Meanwhile mix together coconut flour, parmesan, paprika, garlic powder, onion powder salt and pepper in a bowl.

Dip chicken first in coconut flour mixture then in beaten egg.

Heat avocado oil in a skillet and cook chicken from both sides. Until lightly brown and cooked

Set chicken zinger between two chaffles with lettuce and bbq sauce.

Enjoy!

Nutrition:

Amount per serving 288 g

Total calories 719 kcal

Fats 49.75 g

Protein 53.32 g

Net carbs 8.1 g

Fiber 6 g

Starch 0.21 g

Chaffle & chicken lunch plate

Preparation time: 5 min

Cooking time: 15 min

Servings: 1

Ingredients

1 large egg

1/2 cup jack cheese, shredded

1 pinch salt

For serving

1 chicken leg

Salt

Pepper

1 tsp. Garlic, minced

1 egg

I tsp avocado oil

Directions

Heat your square waffle maker and grease with Cooking spray.

Pour chaffle batter intothe skillet and cook for about 2-3 minutes.

Meanwhile, heat oil in a pan, over medium heat.

Once the oil is hot, add chicken thigh and garlicthen, cook for about 4-5 minutes. Flip and cook for another 3-4 minutes.

Season with salt and pepper and give them a good mix.

Transfer cooked thigh to plate.

Fry the egg in the same pan for about 1-2 minutes according to your choice.

Once chaffles are cooked, Servings with fried egg and chicken thigh.

Enjoy!

Nutrition:

Amount per serving 194 g

Total calories 440 kcal

Fats 32.92 g

Protein 32.11 g

Net carbs 1.77 g

Fiber 0.1 g

Starch 0 g

Grill pork chaffle sandwich

Preparation time: 5 min

Cooking time: 15 min

Servings: 2

Ingredients

1/2 cup mozzarella, shredded

1 egg

I pinch garlic powder

Pork patty

1/2 cup pork, minced

1 tbsp. Green onion, diced

1/2 tsp italian seasoning

Lettuce leaves

Directions

Preheat the square waffle maker and grease with

Mix together egg, cheese and garlic powder in a small mixing bowl.

Pour batter in a preheated waffle maker and close the lid.

Make 2 chaffles from thisbatter.

Cook chaffles for about 2-3 minutes until cooked through.

Meanwhile, mix together pork patty Ingredients in a bowl and make 1 large patty.

Grill pork patty in a preheated grill for about 3-4 minutes per side until cooked through.

Arrange pork patty between two chaffles with lettuce leaves. Cut sandwich to make a triangular sandwich.

Enjoy!

Nutrition:

Amount per serving 95 g

Total calories 181 kcal

Fats 9.58 g

Protein 20.45 g

Net carbs 1.12 g

Fiber 0.1 g

Starch 0 g

Double chicken chaffles

Preparation time: 5 min

Cooking time: 5 min

Servings: 2

Ingredients

1/2 cup boil shredded chicken

1/4 cup cheddar cheese

1/8 cup parmesan cheese

1 egg

1 tsp. Italian seasoning

1/8 tsp. Garlic powder

1 tsp. Cream cheese

Directions

Preheat the belgian waffle maker.

Mix together in chaffle Ingredients in a bowl and mix together.

Sprinkle 1 tbsp. Of cheese in a waffle maker and pour in chaffle batter.

Pour 1 tbsp. Of cheese over batter and close the lid.

Cook chaffles for about 4 to 5 minutes.

Servings with a chicken zinger and enjoy the double chicken flavor.

Nutrition:

Amount per serving 78 g

Total calories 199 kcal

Fats 14.34 g

Protein 14.35 g

Net carbs 1.83 g

Fiber 0.2 g

Starch 0 g

Chicken bites with chaffles

Preparation time 5 min

Cooking time 10 min

Servings: 2

Ingredients: 1 egg, whisked

1 chicken breastscut into 2 x2 inch chunks

1/4 cup almond flour

2 tbsps. Onion powder

2 tbsps. Garlic powder

1 tsp. Dried oregano

1 tsp. Paprika powder 1 tsp. Salt

1/2 tsp. Black pepper

2 tbsps. Avocado oil

Directions

Add all the dry Ingredients together into a large bowl. Mix well. Place the eggs into a separate bowl. Dip each chicken piece into the egg and then into the dry Ingredients. Heat oil in 10-inch skillet, add oil. Once avocado oil is hot, place the coated chicken nuggets onto a skillet and cook for 6-8 minutes until cooked and golden brown.   Servings with chaffles and raspberries. Enjoy!

Nutrition: Amount per serving 173 g

Total calories 401 kcal Fats 28.19 g

Protein 32.35 g Net carbs 1.46 g

Fiber 3 g Starch 0.13 g

Cauliflower chaffles

and tomatoes

Preparation time: 5 min

Cooking time: 15 min

Servings: 2 t

Ingredients

1/2 cup cauliflower

1/4 tsp. Garlic powder

1/4 tsp. Black pepper

1/4 tsp. Salt

1/2 cup shredded cheddar cheese

1 egg

For topping

1 lettuce leave

1 tomato sliced

4 oz. Cauliflower steamed, mashed

1 tsp sesame seeds

Directions

Add all chaffle Ingredients into a blender and mix well.

Sprinkle 1/8 shredded cheese on the waffle maker and pour cauliflower mixture in a preheated waffle maker and sprinkle the rest of the cheese over it.

Cook chaffles for about 4-5 minutes until cooked

For serving, lay lettuce leaves over chaffle top with steamed cauliflower and tomato.

Drizzle sesame seeds on top.

Enjoy!

Nutrition: Amount per serving 149 g

Total calories 198 kcal Fats 14.34 g

Protein 12.74 g Net carbs 1.73 g

Fiber 2 g Starch 0 g

Chaffle with cheese & bacon

Preparation time: 15 min

Cooking time: 15 min

tt

Servings: 2

Ingredients

1 egg

1/2 cup cheddar cheese, shredded

1 tbsp. Parmesan cheese

3/4 tsp coconut flour

1/4 tsp baking powder

1/8 tsp italian seasoning

Pinch of salt

1/4 tsp garlic powder

For topping

1 bacon sliced, cooked and chopped

1/2 cup mozzarella cheese, shredded

1/4 tsp parsley, chopped

Directions

Preheat oven to 400 degrees.

Switch on your mini waffle maker and grease with Cooking spray.

Mix together chaffle Ingredients in a mixing bowl until combined.

Spoon half of the batter in the center of the waffle maker and close the lid. Cook chaffles for about 3-4 minutes until cooked.

Carefully remove chaffles from the maker.

Arrange chaffles in a greased baking tray.

Top with mozzarella cheese, chopped bacon and parsley.

And bake in the oven for 4 -5 minutes.

Once the cheese is melted, remove from the oven.

Servings and enjoy!

Nutrition: Amount per serving 107 g

Total calories 324 kcal

Fats 24.71 g

Protein 22.2 g

Net carbs 0.95 g

Fiber 0.1 g

Starch 0 g

Chaffle mini sandwich

Preparation time: 5 min

Cooking time: t 10 min

Servings: 2

Ingredients 1 large egg

1/8 cup almond flour 1/2 tsp. Garlic powder

3/4 tsp. Baking powder

1/2 cup shredded cheese

Sandwich filling

2 slices deli ham 2 slices tomatoes

1 slice cheddar cheese

Directions

Grease your square waffle maker and preheat it on medium heat. Mix together chaffle Ingredients in a mixing bowl until well combined. Pour batter intoa square waffle and make two chaffles. Once chaffles are cooked, remove from the maker. For a sandwich,arrange deli ham, tomato slice and cheddar cheese between two chaffles. Cut sandwich from the center. Servings and enjoy!

Nutrition: Amount per serving 96 g

Total calories 239 kcal Fats 17.86 g

Protein 17 g

Net carbs 0.95 g

Fiber 0.3 g

Starch 0 g

Chaffles with topping

Preparation time: 5 min

Cooking time: 10 min

Servings: 3

Ingredients 1 large egg

1 tbsp. Almond flour

1 tbsp. Full-fat greek yogurt

1/8 tsp baking powder

1/4 cup shredded swiss cheese

Topping

4oz. Grillprawns

4 oz. Steamed cauliflower mash

1/2 zucchini sliced 3 lettuce leaves

1 tomato, sliced 1 tbsp. Flax seeds

Directions

Make 3 chaffles with the given chaffles Ingredients. For serving, arrange lettuce leaves on each chaffle. Top with zucchini slice, grill prawns, cauliflower mash and a tomato slice.

Drizzle flax seeds on top.

Servings and enjoy!

Nutrition: Amount per serving 112 g

Total calories 158 kcal Fats 8.41 g

Protein 17.31 g Net carbs 1.14 g

Fiber 1.1 g Starch 0 g

Grill beefsteak and chaffle

Preparation time: 5 min

Cooking time: 10 min

Servings: 1

Ingredients 1 beefsteak rib eye

1 tsp salt 1 tsp pepper

1 tbsp. Lime juice 1 tsp garlic

Directions

Prepare your grill for direct heat.

Mix together all spices and rub over beefsteak evenly.

Place the beef on the grill rack over medium heat.

Cover and cook steak for about6 to 8 minutes. Flip and cook for another 4-5 minutes until cooked through.

Servings with Ketogenic simple chaffle and enjoy!

Nutrition:

Amount per serving 177 g

Total calories 538 kcal

Fats 26.97 g

Protein 68.89 g

Net carbs 3.07 g

Fiber 0.8 g

Starch 0 g

Chaffle cheese sandwich

Preparation time: 5 min

Cooking time: 10 min

Servings: 1

Ingredients

2 square Ketogenic chaffle

2 slice cheddar cheese

2 lettuce leaves

Directions

Prepare your oven on 4000 f.

Arrange lettuce leave and cheese slice between chaffles.

Bake in the preheated oven for about 4-5 minutes until cheese is melted.

Once the cheese is melted, remove from the oven.

Servings and enjoy!

Nutrition:

Amount per serving 70 g

Total calories 215 kcal

Fats 16.69 g

Protein 14.42 g

Net carbs 1.28 g

Fiber 0.1 g

Starch 0 g

Chaffle egg sandwich

Preparation time: 5 min

Cooking time: 10 min

Servings: 2

Ingredients

2 mini Ketogenic chaffle

2 slice cheddar cheese

1 egg simple omelet

Directions

Prepare your oven on 4000 f.

Arrange egg omelet and cheese slice between chaffles.

Bake in the preheated oven for about 4-5 minutes until cheese is melted.

Once the cheese is melted, remove from the oven.

Servings and enjoy!

Nutrition: Amount per serving 185 g

Total calories 495 kcal Fats 37.65 g

Protein 34.41 g Net carbs 2.59 g

Fiber 0.2 g Starch 0.01 g

Cauliflower chaffle

Preparation Time: 15 minutes

Servings: 2

Ingredients:

1 egg, lightly beaten

1 cup cauliflower rice

1/2 cup parmesan cheese, shredded

1/2 cup mozzarella cheese, shredded

1 tsp italian seasoning

1/4 tsp garlic powder

1/4 tsp pepper

1/4 tsp salt

Directions:

Preheat your waffle maker.

Add all Ingredients into the blender and blend until smooth.

Spray waffle maker with Cooking spray.

Pour half batter in the hot waffle maker and cook for 4-5 minutes. Repeat with the remaining batter.

Servings and enjoy.

Nutrition: Calories 239 Fat 15.1 g

Carbohydrates 5.1 g Sugar 1.7 g

Protein 21 g Cholesterol 116 mg

Perfect jalapeno chaffle

Preparation Time: 20 minutes

Servings: 6

Ingredients: 3 eggs

1 cup cheddar cheese, shredded

8 oz cream cheese 2 jalapeno peppers, diced

4 bacon slices, cooked and crumbled

1/2 tsp baking powder 3 tbsp coconut flour

1/4 tsp sea salt

Directions:

Preheat your waffle maker. In a small bowl, mix coconut flour, baking powder, and salt. In a medium bowl, beat cream cheese using a hand mixer until fluffy. In a large bowl, beat eggs until fluffy. Add cheddar cheese and half cup cream in eggs and beat until well combined. Add coconut flour mixture to egg mixture and mix until combined. Add jalapeno pepper and stir well. Spray waffle maker with Cooking spray. Pour 1/4 cup batter in the hot waffle maker and cook for 4-5 minutes. Repeat with the remaining batter. Once chaffle is slightly cool then top with remaining cream cheese and bacon.

Servings and enjoy.

Nutrition: Calories 340 Fat 28 g

Carbohydrates 6.2 g Sugar 1 g

Protein 16.1 g Cholesterol 157 mg

Crunchy zucchini chaffle

Preparation Time: 20 minutes

Servings: 8

Ingredients:

2 eggs, lightly beaten

1 garlic clove, minced

1 1/2 tbsp onion, minced

1 cup cheddar cheese, grated

1 small zucchini, grated and squeeze out all liquid

Directions:

Preheat your waffle maker.

In a bowl, mix eggs, garlic, onion, zucchini, and cheese until well combined.

Spray waffle maker with Cooking spray.

Pour 1/4 cup batter in the hot waffle maker and cook for 5 minutes or until golden brown. Repeat with the remaining batter.

Servings and enjoy.

Nutrition:

Calories 76

Fat 5.8 g

Carbohydrates 1.1 g

Sugar 0.5 g

Protein 5.1 g

Cholesterol 56 mg

Simple cheese bacon chaffles

Preparation Time: 15 minutes

Servings: 4

Ingredients:

2 eggs, lightly beaten

1/4 tsp garlic powder

2 bacon slices, cooked and chopped

3/4 cup cheddar cheese, shredded

Directions:

Preheat your mini waffle maker and spray with Cooking spray.

In a bowl, mix eggs, garlic powder, bacon, and cheese.

Pour 2 tbsp of the batter in the hot waffle maker and cook for 2-3 minutes or until set. Repeat with the remaining batter.

Servings and enjoy.

Nutrition:

Calories 169

Fat 13.2 g

Carbohydrates 0.7 g

Sugar 0.3 g

Protein 11.6 g

Cholesterol 115 mg

Cheddar cauliflower chaffle

Preparation Time: 13 minutes

Servings: 1

Ingredients:

1 egg, lightly beaten

1 tbsp almond flour

1/4 cup cheddar cheese, shredded

1/2 cup cauliflower rice

Pepper

Salt

Directions:

Preheat your waffle maker.

Add all Ingredients into the bowl and mix until well combined.

Spray waffle maker with Cooking spray.

Pour batter in the hot waffle maker and cook for 8 minutes or until golden brown.

Servings and enjoy.

Nutrition:

Calories 230

Fat 17.3 g

Carbohydrates 4.9 g

Sugar 1.9 g

Protein 15.1 g

Cholesterol 193 mg

Ketogenic breakfast chaffle

Preparation Time: 15 minutes

Servings: 2

Ingredients:

1 egg, lightly beaten

½ cup mozzarella cheese, shredded

½ tsp psyllium husk powder

¼ tsp garlic powder

Directions:

Preheat your waffle maker.

Whisk egg in a bowl with remaining Ingredients until well combined.

Spray waffle maker with Cooking spray.

Pour 1/2 of batter in the hot waffle maker and cook until golden brown. Repeat with the remaining batter.

Servings and enjoy.

Nutrition:

Calories 55

Fat 3.4 g

Carbohydrates 1.3 g

Sugar 0.3 g

Protein 4.8 g

Cholesterol 86 mg

Perfect Ketogenic chaffle

Preparation Time: 15 minutes

Servings: 2

Ingredients: 2 eggs, lightly beaten

1/2 cup mozzarella cheese, shredded

1/2 cup cheddar cheese, shredded

1/4 tsp baking powder, gluten-free

1 tbsp almond flour

1/4 tsp cinnamon

1/4 tsp red chili flakes

1/4 tsp salt

Directions:

Preheat your waffle maker and spray with Cooking spray.

In a bowl, whisk eggs with baking powder, almond flour, and salt.

Add remaining Ingredients and mix until well combined.

Pour half of the batter in the hot waffle maker and cook for 3-5 minutes or until golden brown. Repeat with the remaining batter.

Servings and enjoy.

Nutrition: Calories 218

Fat 16.7 g Carbohydrates 2.2 g

Sugar 0.6 g Protein 15.3 g

Cholesterol 197 mg

Cabbage chaffle

Preparation Time: 15 minutes

Servings: 2

Ingredients:

1 egg, lightly beaten

1/3 cup mozzarella cheese, grated

½ bacon slice, chopped

1 ½ tbsp green onion, sliced

2 tbsp cabbage, chopped

2 tbsp almond flour

Pepper

Salt

Directions:

Add all Ingredients in a bowl and stir to combine.

Spray waffle maker with Cooking spray.

Pour half of the batter in the hot waffle maker and cook until golden brown. Repeat with the remaining batter.

Servings and enjoy.

Nutrition: Calories 113

Fat 8.5 g Carbohydrates 2.5 g

Sugar 0.7 g Protein 7.5 g

Cholesterol 90 mg

Simple ham chaffle

Preparation Time: 15 minutes

Servings: 2

Ingredients: 1 egg, lightly beaten

1/4 cup ham, chopped

1/2 cup cheddar cheese, shredded

1/4 tsp garlic salt

For dip:

1 1/2 tsp dijon mustard

1 tbsp mayonnaise

Directions:

Preheat your waffle maker.

Whisk eggs in a bowl.

Stir in ham, cheese, and garlic salt until combine.

Spray waffle maker with Cooking spray.

Pour half of the batter in the hot waffle maker and cook for 3-4 minutes or until golden brown. Repeat with the remaining batter.

For dip: in a small bowl, mix mustard and mayonnaise. Servings chaffle with dip.

Nutrition: Calories 205 Fat 15.6 g

Carbohydrates 3.4 g

Sugar 0.9 g Protein 12.9 g

Cholesterol 123 mg

Delicious bagel chaffle

Preparation Time: 15 minutes

Servings: 2

Ingredients:

1 egg, lightly beaten

1/4 tsp garlic powder

1/4 tsp onion powder

1 1/2 tsp bagel seasoning

3/4 cup mozzarella cheese, shredded

1/2 tsp baking powder, gluten-free

1 tbsp almond flour

Directions:

Preheat your waffle maker.

In a bowl, mix egg, bagel seasoning, baking powder, onion powder, garlic powder, and almond flour until well combined.

Add cheese and stir well.

Spray waffle maker with Cooking spray.

Pour 1/2 of batter in the hot waffle maker and cook for 5 minutes or until golden brown. Repeat with the remaining batter.

Servings and enjoy.

Nutrition: Calories 85 Fat 5.8 g

Carbohydrates 2.4 g Sugar 0.5 g

Protein 6.6 g Cholesterol 87 mg

Cheesy garlic bread chaffle

Preparation Time: 15 minutes

Servings: 2

Ingredients: 1 egg, lightly beaten

1 tsp parsley, minced

2 tbsp parmesan cheese, grated

1 tbsp butter, melted

1/4 tsp garlic powder

1/4 tsp baking powder, gluten-free

1 tsp coconut flour

1/2 cup cheddar cheese, shredded

Directions:

Preheat your waffle maker. In a bowl, whisk egg, garlic powder, baking powder, coconut flour, and cheddar cheese until well combined. Spray waffle maker with Cooking spray. Pour half of the batter in the hot waffle maker and cook for 3 minutes or until set. Repeat with the remaining batter.

Brush chaffles with melted butter.

Place chaffles on baking tray and top with parmesan cheese and broil until cheese melted.

Garnish with parsley and Servings.

Nutrition: Calories 248 Fat 19.4 g

Carbohydrates 5.4 g Sugar 1 g

Protein 12.5 g Cholesterol 131 mg

Zucchini basil chaffle

Preparation Time: 15 minutes

Servings: 2

Ingredients: 1 egg, lightly beaten

1/4 cup fresh basil, chopped

1/4 cup mozzarella cheese, shredded

1/2 cup parmesan cheese, shredded

1 cup zucchini, grated and squeeze out all liquid

1/4 tsp pepper

3/4 tsp salt

Directions:

Preheat your waffle maker.

In a small bowl, beat the egg.

Add basil, mozzarella cheese, zucchini, pepper, and salt and stir well.

Spray waffle maker with Cooking spray.

Sprinkle 2 tbsp of parmesan cheese to the bottom of waffle iron then spread 1/4 of the batter and top with 2 tbsp parmesan cheese and cook for 4-8 minutes or until set. Repeat with the remaining batter.

Servings and enjoy.

Nutrition: Calories 218 Fat 13.9 g

Carbohydrates 3.8 g Sugar 1.2 g

Protein 19.7 g Cholesterol 113 mg

Jicama chaffle

Preparation Time: 15 minutes

Servings: 2

Ingredients:

2 eggs, lightly beaten

1 cup cheddar cheese, shredded

1/4 tsp garlic powder

1/4 tsp onion powder

1 large jicama root, peel, shredded and squeeze out all liquid

Pepper

Salt

Directions:

Preheat your waffle maker. Add shredded jicama in microwave-safe bowl and microwave for 5-8 minutes.

Add remaining Ingredients to the bowl and stir to combine.

Spray waffle maker with Cooking spray.

Pour half of the batter in the hot waffle maker and cook until golden brown or set. Repeat with the remaining batter.

Servings and enjoy.

Nutrition: Calories 315

Fat 23.1 g Carbohydrates 7.1 g

Sugar 2.3 g Protein 20.2 g

Cholesterol 223 mg

Tasty broccoli chaffle

Preparation Time: 15 minutes

Servings: 3

Ingredients:

2 eggs, lightly beaten

1/3 cup parmesan cheese, grated

1 cup cheddar cheese, shredded

1 cup broccoli

Directions:

Preheat your waffle maker.

Add broccoli into the food processor and process until it looks like rice. Transfer broccoli into the mixing bowl.

Add remaining Ingredients into the bowl and mix until well combined.

Spray waffle maker with Cooking spray.

Pour 1/3 of batter in the hot waffle maker and cook for 4-5 minutes until golden brown. Repeat with the remaining batter.

Servings and enjoy.

Nutrition: Calories 271

Fat 19.5 g Carbohydrates 2.7 g

Sugar 1 g Protein 19.3 g

Cholesterol 162 mg

Quick carnivore chaffle

Preparation Time: 10 minutes

Servings: 1

Ingredients:

1 egg, lightly beaten

1/3 cup cheddar cheese, shredded

1/2 cup ground pork rinds

Pinch of salt

Directions:

Preheat your waffle maker.

In a bowl, whisk egg, pork rinds, cheese, and salt.

Spray waffle maker with Cooking spray.

Pour batter in the hot waffle maker and cook for 5 minutes until golden brown.

Servings and enjoy.

Nutrition:

Calories 275

Fat 20.2 g

Carbohydrates 0.8 g

Sugar 0.5 g

Protein 23.6 g

Cholesterol 203 mg

Cinnamon chaffle

Preparation Time: 15 minutes

Servings: 2

Ingredients:

1 egg, lightly beaten

1/2 tsp vanilla

1/2 tsp cinnamon

1/2 cup mozzarella cheese, shredded

Directions:

Preheat your waffle maker.

In a small bowl, whisk egg, vanilla, cinnamon, and cheese until well combined.

Spray waffle maker with Cooking spray.

Pour half batter in the hot waffle maker and cook until golden brown. Repeat with the remaining batter.

Servings and enjoy.

Nutrition:

Calories 56

Fat 3.5 g

Carbohydrates 1 g

Sugar 0.3 g

Protein 4.8 g

Cholesterol 86 mg

Ketogenic Breakfast Chaffle

Preparation time: 3 *Minutes*

Cooking Time : 6 *Minutes*

Servings: 1

Ingredients: 2 tablespoons butter

1 egg 1/2 cup Monterey Jack Cheese

1 tablespoon almond flour

Directions

Preheat mini waffle maker until hot

Whisk egg in a bowl, add cheese, then mix well

Stir in the remaining Ingredients (except toppings, if any).

Grease waffle maker and Scoop 1/2 of the batter onto the waffle maker, spread across evenly

Cook until a bit browned and crispy, about 4 minutes.

Gently remove from waffle maker and let it cool

Repeat with remaining batter.

Melt butter in a pan. Add chaffles to the pan and cook for 2 minutes on each side

Remove from the pan and let it cool.

Servings and Enjoy!

Nutrition: 257 calories 1g net carbs 24g fat 11g protein

Pumpkin chaffle

Preparation time: 5 minutes

Cooking time: 5 minutes

Servings: 2

Ingredients:

½ cup mozzarella cheese, shredded

1 tablespoon coconut flour

1 egg, whisked

1 tablespoon stevia

2 tablespoons pumpkin puree

2 tablespoons cream cheese

½ teaspoon almond extract

Directions:

In a bowl, mix the mozzarella with the flour, egg and the other Ingredients and whisk well.

Heat up the waffle iron over high heat, pour half of the batter, close the waffle maker, cook for 5 minutes and transfer to a plate.

Repeat with the other part of the batter and Servings the chaffles warm.

Nutrition: calories 200, fat 15, fiber 1.2, carbs 3.4, protein 12.05

Carrot cake chaffles

Preparation time: 10 minutes

Cooking time: 10 minutes

Servings: 4

Ingredients:

2 tablespoons cream cheese, soft

½ cup carrots, peeled and grated

2 tablespoons stevia

1 egg, whisked

½ teaspoon baking powder

3 tablespoons almond flour

½ cup heavy cream

1 tablespoon swerve

Directions:

In a bowl, mix the carrots with the cream cheese and the other Ingredients except the heavy cream and swerve whisk.

Heat up the waffle iron, divide the batter into 4 parts and cook the chaffles.

In a bowl mix the heavy cream with the swerve and whisk.

Layer the chaffles and the cream and Servings the cake cold.

Nutrition: calories 251, fat 13, fiber 2.3, carbs 5, protein 6

Italian garlic chaffle

Preparation Time: 15 minutes

Servings: 2

Ingredients:

1 egg, lightly beaten

1/8 tsp italian seasoning

1/4 tsp garlic, minced

1/4 cup parmesan cheese, grated

1/2 cup mozzarella cheese, shredded

Directions:

Preheat your waffle maker.

In a small bowl, whisk egg, italian seasoning, garlic, parmesan cheese, and mozzarella cheese until well combined.

Spray waffle maker with Cooking spray.

Pour half batter in the hot waffle maker and cook for 4-5 minutes or until golden brown. Repeat with the remaining batter.

Servings and enjoy.

Nutrition:

Calories 128 Fat 8 g

Carbohydrates 0.6 g

Sugar 0.2 g

Protein 10.8 g

Cholesterol 101 mg

Tuna dill chaffle

Preparation Time: 15 minutes

Servings: 2

Ingredients:

1 egg, lightly beaten

1 dill pickle, sliced

1 tbsp mayonnaise

1/3 cup cheddar cheese, shredded

1 can tuna, drained

Directions:

Preheat your waffle maker.

Add all Ingredients in mixing bowl and whisk until well combined.

Spray waffle maker with Cooking spray.

Pour half batter in the hot waffle maker and cook for 5 minutes. Repeat with the remaining batter.

Servings and enjoy.

Nutrition:

Calories 305

Fat 18.1 g

Carbohydrates 2.9 g

Sugar 1.1 g

Protein 31.3 g

Cholesterol 131 mg

Perfect breakfast chaffle

Preparation Time: 15 minutes

Servings: 2

Ingredients: 1 egg, lightly beaten

1/2 tsp baking powder, gluten-free

1 tbsp almond flour

1/4 cup mozzarella cheese, shredded

1/4 cup cheddar cheese, shredded

1/4 tsp onion powder

1/4 tsp garlic powder

1/4 tsp cinnamon

Pepper

Salt

Directions:

Preheat your waffle maker.

Add all Ingredients into the mixing bowl and mix well.

Spray waffle maker with Cooking spray.

Pour half batter in the hot waffle maker and cook until golden brown. Repeat with the remaining batter.

Servings and enjoy.

Nutrition: Calories 123

Fat 9.3 g Carbohydrates 2.6 g

Sugar 0.6 g Protein 8.2 g Cholesterol 99 mg

Coconut scallion chaffle

Preparation Time: 15 minutes

Servings: 2

Ingredients:

1 egg, lightly beaten

1 ½ tsp coconut flour

2 tbsp scallions, sliced

1 cup cheddar cheese, shredded

1 cup mozzarella cheese, shredded

Pepper

Salt

Directions:

Preheat your waffle maker.

Add all Ingredients in a bowl and mix well.

Spray waffle maker with Cooking spray.

Pour half batter in the hot waffle maker and cook until golden brown. Repeat with the remaining batter.

Servings and enjoy.

Nutrition:

Calories 346 Fat 24.9 g

Carbohydrates 7.9 g

Sugar 1.4 g Protein 22.5 g

Cholesterol 149 mg

Jalapeno ham chaffle

Preparation Time: 20 minutes

Servings: 4

Ingredients:

2 eggs, lightly beaten

2 tsp coconut flour

1 tbsp green onion, chopped

2 oz ham, chopped

1/2 jalapeno pepper, grated

2 oz cheddar cheese, shredded

Directions:

Preheat your waffle maker.

Add all Ingredients into the mixing bowl and mix until well combined.

Spray waffle maker with Cooking spray.

Pour 1/4 of the batter in the hot waffle maker and cook for 3-4 minutes or until golden brown. Repeat with the remaining batter.

Servings and enjoy.

Nutrition:

Calories 143 Fat 9.1 g Carbohydrates 5.1 g

Sugar 0.8 g Protein 9.7 g

Cholesterol 105 mg

Tasty jalapeno chaffle

Preparation Time: 10 minutes

Servings: 1

Ingredients:

1 egg, lightly beaten

1 tbsp olive oil

1 tbsp jalapeno, chopped

1 tbsp almond flour

1/2 cup cheddar cheese, shredded

Directions:

Preheat your waffle maker.

Add all Ingredients into the bowl and whisk until well combined.

Spray waffle maker with Cooking spray.

Pour batter in the hot waffle maker and cook until golden brown.

Servings and enjoy.

Nutrition:

Calories 465

Fat 43.9 g

Carbohydrates 4.2 g

Sugar 0.8 g

Protein 21.1 g

Cholesterol 234 mg

Crispy chaffle

Preparation Time: 15 minutes

Servings: 4

Ingredients:

2 eggs, lightly beaten

1 cup cheddar cheese, shredded

1/4 tsp baking powder, gluten-free

1/4 cup almond flour

Directions:

Preheat your waffle maker and spray with Cooking spray.

In a bowl, whisk eggs, baking powder, and almond flour.

Add cheese and stir to combine.

Pour 1/4 of the batter in the hot waffle maker and cook until golden brown. Repeat with the remaining batter.

Servings and enjoy.

Nutrition:

Calories 186

Fat 15.1 g

Carbohydrates 2.2 g

Sugar 0.6 g

Protein 11.3 g

Cholesterol 112 mg

Crispy cheddar cheese chaffle

Preparation Time: 13 minutes

Servings: 1

Ingredients:

1 egg, lightly beaten

2 oz cheddar cheese, thinly sliced

Directions:

Preheat your waffle maker and spray with Cooking spray.

Arrange half cheese slices on hot waffle maker then pour the egg on top.

Now place remaining cheese slices on top and cook for 6-8 minutes.

Servings and enjoy.

Nutrition:

Calories 291

Fat 23.2 g

Carbohydrates 1.1 g

Sugar 0.6 g

Protein 19.7 g

Cholesterol 223 mg

Berry chaffle

Preparation time: 5 minutes

Cooking time: 5 minutes

Servings: 2

Ingredien ts:

1 egg, whisked

2 tablespoons stevia

1 teaspoon coconut flour

4 strawberries, chopped

½ teaspoon baking powder

1 teaspoon cream cheese, soft

Directions:

In a bowl, mix the berries with the egg, stevia and the other Ingredients and whisk well.

Heat up the waffle iron over medium-high heat, pour half of the batter, close the waffle maker, cook for 5 minutes and transfer to a plate.

Repeat with the other half of the batter and Servings the chaffles warm.

Nutrition: calories 58, fat 5, fiber 1.2, carbs 2, protein 3.2

Cinnamon chaffle

Preparation time: 5 minutes

Cooking time: 5 minutes

Servings: 1

Ingredients:

Cooking spray

2 ounces cream cheese, soft 1 egg, whisked

2 teaspoons monk fruit sweetener

1 teaspoon coconut flour

2 teaspoons cinnamon powder

½ teaspoon baking soda

Directions:

In a bowl, mix the cream cheese with the egg and the other Ingredients except the Cooking spray and whisk well.

Grease the waffle iron with the Cooking spray, pour the batter, spread, close the waffle maker, cook for 5 minutes, transfer to a plate and Servings.

Nutrition: calories 121, fat 8.4, fiber 2.3, carbs 4, protein 2.3